# Aging Ant

*The Ultimate Key to Achieving Longevity*

*Naturally*

## Shayne Perry

ISBN: 978-1-63750-045-3

# Table of Contents

# Introduction

An exceptional book from one of Time's Most Influential People, Shayne Perry. It is an undeniable fact that Aging is inevitable. But what happens if all we learned about it is not correct? What if we could determine how long we would live (lifespan).

In this paradigm-shifting book, Shayne Perry, a leading authority in genetics and longevity, exposes a new gigantic theory about the reason we age. As he once said, "aging is a disease, and the disease can be treated."

This book is an eye-opener that reveals many incredible breakthroughs that demonstrate how we can reverse and also slow down aging. He aims at activating practices and lifestyle changes that is both the cause and key to reversing aging.

A recent research in genetic engineering proposes that in the near future, we won't just feel younger, but actually become more youthful.

In a narrative research work, Shayne Perry, reveals the discovery of natural and lifestyle changes such as exercising, intermittent fasting, eating whole foods, eating less meat and more plant-based foods; that have been shown to help humans to live longer, healthier and feel younger. We have to take charge of our own health and that of the generation after us and, for the future of humanity. Humanity will forever be grateful for this discovery, their thought about aging will change and the lasting solution will be utilized for generations

# Chapter 1

## Aging Overview

### The Facts

Everybody knows the obvious signs of aging which are lines and wrinkles, grey hair, a slightly stooped posture, perhaps, some "senior occasions" of forgetfulness...etc. Have you ever asked yourself why all these happen? This question leads us to what aging really entails. Each person comprises cellular materials of about 13 trillion. Our cells and organs both constitute the cellular materials that are held as well as the various natural materials that the cellular material has made.

As soon as conception sets in, our cells, tissues, and organs begin an activity of aging. Premature in life, of course, we are growing, and growing the number of cells that people have. The cellular material also ages but so somewhat that people can't view it. We just start to see the body growing and developing.

Sooner or later in life, often in the '30s, the tell-tale signs of aging start to be apparent. They could be seen in vital symptoms (like blood circulation pressure) to your skin, to your muscle and bones, to your cardiovascular, digestive, and nervous systems and beyond. Some Aging changes start prematurely in life, for instance, your metabolism begins to gradually decrease starting at about age 20. Changes in your hearing, on the other hand, do not usually start until the age range of 50 years and above.

We do not yet grasp the organic interplay of factors that cause us to age, once we do, we would realize that various things impact Aging like genetics, diet, exercise, disease, and a bunch of other factors that give rise to growing older.

Some remarkable biological clinical tests carried out in the 1990s were able to recognize genes that could profoundly influence the pace at which cells and animals age. The good thing from these studies is that natural changes that lengthen life also appear to increase vitality. Pets that live much longer stay quite healthy for the majority of their lengthened life.

None of the discoveries is near to providing an "elixir of youth" for humans, however, many scientists think that research breakthroughs regarding maturity in the 21st hundred years will lead to the introduction of drugs that can extend human beings' life and simultaneously improve individual health. If that occurs, of course, it'll only be considered a positive thing if the world discovers room, work, and resources for all the additional people.

The following are the ways Aging affects a few of our major body systems.

**Cells, Organs, and Tissue:**

- Cellular material becomes less in a position to divide

- The telomeres at the ends of the chromosomes inside every cell gradually get shorter until the cellular dies

- Waste materials accumulate

- The connective tissue between your cells becomes stiffer

- The maximum functional capacity of several organs decreases

**Heart and arteries:**

- The wall of the heart gets thicker.

- The heart muscle becomes less efficient (working significantly harder to pump the same number of the blood)

- The aorta (your body's main artery) becomes thicker, stiffer, and less flexible.

- Lots of the body's arteries including arteries offering  blood to the cardiovascular and brain slowly develop atherosclerosis, although the problem never becomes severe in a few people

**Vital signals:**

- It is harder for the body to control its temperature

- Heart rate takes longer to come back on track after exercise

**Bones, muscles, joint parts:**

- Bones become thinner and less strong

- Joint become stiffer and less flexible

- The cartilage and bone in joints starts to weaken

- Muscle mass becomes less bulky and less strong

**Digestive tract:**

- The movement of food through the digestive tract becomes slower.

- The stomach, liver organ, pancreas, and small intestine make small numbers of digestive juices

**Brain and nervous system:**

- The number of nerve cells in the mind and spinal-cord decreases.

- The number of connections between nerve cells decreases.

- Abnormal structures known as plaques and tangles may form in the mind.

**Eyes and Ear:**

- The retinas get thinner, the irises get stiffer.

- The lens becomes less clear.

- The walls of the ear canal get thinner.

- The eardrums get thicker

**Skin, fingernails, and  hair:**

- Skin gets thinner and becomes less elastic.

- Sweat glands produce less sweat.

- Fingernails grow more slowly.

- Hairs get grey and stop to grow

# Meaning of Aging

*What is Aging?*

Think of Aging as "whatever happens to your bodies as time passes." This description encompasses all the aging the body goes through, instead of the indicators of aging that happen later in life, like grey hair and lines and wrinkles.

Changes which bring about aging are caused by your body. Think of kids growing and teens going right through puberty; Aging also accumulates as time passes, like damaged skin surface triggered by sun exposure. As a result of this, Aging is a mixture of physical changes and the impact of how exactly we look after ourselves.

In other words, aging is the impact of your time on your body, and it occurs in multiple quantities:

- Cellular aging. Cellular material is predicated on the number of times it has replicated. A cell can replicate about 50 times provided that the hereditary material is no more in a position to be copied accurately, which is because of shortened telomeres. The greater the harm done to cellular materials by free radicals and other factors, the greater the cells need to reproduce.

- Hormonal aging: The hormones in the body play enormous factors in Aging, especially during childhood development and adolescent maturity. Hormone quantity fluctuates through life. Puberty brings acne and bigger pores. Once we get older, hormone changes lead to dry pores, dry skin, and menopause.

- Accumulated damage: Accumulated harm is all exterior. Exposure to harmful toxins, the sun, dangerous foods, air pollution, and smoke have a toll on your body. As time passes, these exterior factors can result in injury and your body falls behind in its capability to keep up and repair cellular material, cells, and organs.

- Metabolic Aging: As you start your entire day, your cellular materials are constantly turning food into energy which produces byproducts that may be harmful. The procedure of metabolizing and creating energy leads to damage to your body as time passes. Some think that slowing the fat burning capacity through methods such as calorie limitation may slow Aging in humans.

## Aging Doesn't Discriminate

Our age-obsessed culture is totally consumed with slowing aging and increasing longevity but Aging is completely unavoidable. Growing older doesn't discriminate. It begins premature and it impacts every major body organ in the torso.

For instance, around the time one is twenty years old, lung cells lose their elasticity, the muscles around the rib cage start to deteriorate and lung function, that is, the quantity of air that may be inhaled, lowers. Creation of digestive enzymes decreases, which impacts how nutrients are absorbed into the body.

Fatty deposits build up in the arteries at the center and the vessels begin to lose versatility, leading to atherosclerosis or the hardening of the arteries. In women, genital fluid production reduces and sexual tissue atrophy occur. For men, the prostate may become enlarged and sperm creation decreases.

# Chapter 2

## Diagnosis

Although your body and mind proceed through many natural changes even as you age, not absolutely all changes are normal. There are numerous misconceptions in what is a standard part of Aging. Senility, for example, is not really a natural consequence of getting old though many people think it is.

It's important to speak to your doctor about any changes you are experiencing. Your physician will help you differentiate between what is a normal part of Aging and what's not. If required, your physician may send you to an expert.

## Symptoms

We each age at different rates and also to different degrees, yet we experience many common effects of aging. Some typically common signs or symptoms of Aging include:

- Increased susceptibility to infection.

- Greater threat of warmth stroke or hypothermia.

- A slight reduction in elevation as the bone fragments of our spines get thinner and lose some height.

- Bones break easier.

- Joint changes range from small stiffness to severe arthritis.

- Stooped posture.

- Slow and limited movement.

- Reduction in overall energy.

- Constipation.

- Urinary incontinence.

- Minor slowing of thought, memory space, and pondering (however, delirium, dementia, and severe storage loss aren't a standard part of aging).

- Slow response to reflexes, reduction in coordination and difficulty in body balancing.

- Reduction in visual acuity.

- Reduced peripheral vision.

- Some extent of hearing loss.

- Wrinkling and sagging skin.

- Whitening or graying of hair.

- Weight reduction after age 55 in men and after age 65 in women partly due to lack of muscle tissue.

## Expected Duration

Aging is a continuing, progressive process that continues until the end of life.

# Chapter 3

## Prevention of Premature Aging

We cannot change our genes nor stop the duration of time. However, through changes in lifestyle, we can reduce our risk for a few of the diseases and conditions that are more coming once we age. We are able to also ward off diseases with screening assessments and immunizations

**Screening tests**; tests can identify diseases prematurely, and possibly curative, phases. However, the benefits of csreening tests and methods drop as you grow older. Indeed, testing tests will often lead to damage. For instance, if the test is falsely positive, screening may be purchased.

Work with your physician to determine whether you ought to have a particular test. For instance, a test for a specific disease might not be necessary if your threat of getting that disease is surprisingly low, to begin with. Or if you understand you'll not acknowledge treatment for a specific disease, if it was found out by verification test, then it could not be well worth getting the test to begin with. Or if it could not expand or improve your life to find and treat a specific disease, then it could not be worthy of doing a test for the condition. Only your medical provider and you may determine whether tests are advantageous.

Immunizations; in 2014, the U.S Centers for Disease Control and Avoidance suggested that adults have the next immunizations

- Influenza, each year;

- Pneumococcal pneumonia vaccine, if in the 19-64 a long time with risk for pneumococcal infection (such as from persistent heart or lung disease), with least one immunization for everybody after age 65;

- Tetanus, diphtheria, and pertussis (one-shot using one occasion), and then tetanus and diphtheria every decade;

- Varicella (the virus that triggers chickenpox and zoster, also known as shingles), if you didn't understand this vaccine as a kid.

- Herpes zoster (shingles) vaccine for individual's ages 60 and over, even if indeed they experienced an assault of shingles earlier in life.

- Meningococcal vaccine, if you are in particular risk because of this condition (speak to your doctor);

- Human papillomavirus vaccine, if you're between the age 19-26 (people who get the vaccine at age 19-21 require it again at 22-26 a long time if they're at risk of this infection, such as when sexually. Hepatitis A disease and hepatitis B malware vaccines, if you didn't have them as a kid, and if you are a specific risk because of this infection.

- Hemophilic influenza type B vaccine, if you are at risk of this infection.

These are general suggestions for older adults. For a few old adults, additional immunizations may be suggested. For others, such as people who have weakened defense systems, some generally suggested immunizations shouldn't be given. To type this all out, talk to your doctor.

## Treatment

As you age, it's important to take into account not only how long you will live, but how well you will live. The next strategies can help you keep up as well as perhaps even improve your standard of living as you age.

- Don't smoke cigarettes: Smoking plays a part in cardiovascular disease, osteoporosis, and heart stroke, and it does increase the risk of several malignancies. Smoking even seems to make someone's memory worse. The good tidings are that individuals who stop smoking can repair some, if not absolutely all, of the harm done by many years of smoking.

- Build physical and mental activities into every day: Exercise is wonderful for your body and your brain. Exercise and even activity such as gardening or housekeeping help maintain your bone fragments and healthy heart, as well as your weight in balance. Studies also have shown that actually energetic people lower their risk of developing dementia and will stay mentally energetic. And staying psychologically active helps defend against memory loss.

- Eating a healthy diet rich in whole grains, vegetables, and fruits, and alternative healthier monounsaturated and polyunsaturated fats instead of harmful fats and Trans fats. Such a diet plan protects you against many diseases, like heart disease, malignancy, and stroke.

- Have a daily multivitamin, and make sure to get enough calcium and vitamin D. This means 1200 milligrams (mg) of calcium each day for women and men age 50 years and older. Daily vitamin D recommendations range between 600 IU each day for adults under age 60 and 600-1,000 IU each day for individuals over age group 60. An increasing number of experts recommend up to at least 1,000 IU every day, although the worthiness of this is not proved by scientific tests.

- Maintain a healthy weight and body shape. As we grow older, our metabolism slows, which makes it harder to melt calories. But extra bodyweight can boost the risk of cardiovascular disease, diabetes, stroke, and certain malignancies. The body form is important as well. Women and men who carry more excess weight around their abdomens have an increased risk of coronary attack and heart stroke than those who bring additional weight around their sides.

- Challenge your brain; some evidence shows that reading, doing crossword puzzles, playing the drum, even participating in mind-provoking discussions, can help to keep your mind razor-sharp.

- Create a strong social network; as you grow older, it is critical to maintaining close and rewarding ties with relatives and buddies and also to create new contacts when possible. Some studies claim that sociable ties will help defend against dementia and keep you environmentally sharpened. Other studies claim that strong cultural connections can help your home is longer.

- Protect your sight, hearing, and health and wellness by pursuing preventive care and attention guidelines.

- Floss, clean, and visit a dental professional regularly. Poor teeth health may have many repercussions, including poor nourishment, unnecessary pain, and perhaps a higher threat of cardiovascular disease and stroke.

- Discuss with your physician whether you will need any medication to regulate high blood pressure, treat osteoporosis, or lower cholesterol to help you remain healthy.

## Slowing of Aging Processes

As mentioned, aging cannot be avoided but there are however several steps you can take to aid your biological clock and help you live longer during this aging period. These include;

- **Eating well**: For the past recent decades, processed food items have become an extremely bigger part of our diets. Added sugars, salt, and excess fat are wreaking havoc on our anatomies, leading to a variety of serious medical issues, including coronary disease and hypertension. Be kind to yourself and eat well. Read brands. Cut out sweet drinks and white starches and incorporate more fruits, vegetables, dietary fiber, and lean protein.

- **No Smoking**: If you are a cigarette smoker, you have to deliberately and intentionally give up on smoking to enhance effective blood circulation, blood pressure and significantly minimizes your risk of developing cancer.

- **Exercise**: You might possibly not be able to do the recommended thirty minutes of the exercise activity each day, however, the very good news is that even just quarter-hour of moderate activity per day can improve durability, for instance, you can walk your dog, trip a bicycle or have a fitness course. Any activity is preferable to none.

- **Socializing**: Socialization keeps us young and well for a long life. Maintain good and healthy associations with others. Stay linked to the ones you love and make it a spot to meet new people.

- **Sleeping well**: Pay a lesser emphasis on the common saying that only a lazy man sleeps too much at night, have a lovely night rest every evening and you'll lessen your risk of having cardiovascular disease and also the rate at which you stress yourself should be reduced drastically.

- **Avoidance of unnecessary stress:** Stress, anger, and, keeping of grudges can be quite emotionally damaging, hence, for the sake of a good health, it is advisable that all these are avoided, instead of allowing these to weigh you down, you can get yourself engaged in positive activities that you enjoy doing thereby eradicating the constitution of unnecessary stress which can mar your heart, also always create a break period for yourself in the course of your daily work.

# Chapter 4

## Premature Aging

*Facts to consider*

As you grow older, your body's internal processes from epidermis cellular turnover to workout recovery decelerate and take much longer to complete or recharge.

This leaves room for signs of aging, such as wrinkles and fatigue, which occur. These changes may be surprising if indeed they happen sooner than expected, hence the word "premature" aging.

It's impossible to avoid these changes completely, but there are ways to lessen the indicators of aging within you particularly if they're happening before you're prepared to embrace them.

Here are things to watch out for, why it happens, and more.

## Causes premature aging

There are always a few different factors that have a direct

impact on how quickly these signs appear on the body.

- **Smoking**

The toxins in tobacco smoke expose your skin layer to oxidative stress. This causes dryness, lines and wrinkles, and other symptoms of premature Aging.

- **Sun exposure and tanning**

Tanning mattresses and contact with the sun permeate your skin layer with Ultra violet rays. These rays harm the DNA in your skin layer cells, causing lines and wrinkles.

- **Genes**

There are a few very rare genetic conditions that can make you show signs of aging in childhood and premature puberty. These conditions are called progeria.

Werner syndrome impacts 1 in 1 million people. It causes wrinkled epidermis, graying locks, and balding to build up between 13 and 30 years old.

Hutchinson-Gilford syndrome can be an even rarer

condition, influencing 1 in 8 million infants.

Children with these symptoms don't develop as quickly as others in their age group. In addition, they experience slim limbs and hair loss. The average life span for children coping with Hutchinson-Gilford symptoms is 13 years.

## Are there other factors?

Several lifestyle habits can contribute to how quickly the body shows signals of Aging, even if indeed they aren't an initial cause.

- **Sleep habits**

Sleep gives the body a chance to refresh and regenerate cellular material.

At least one study has indicated that poor rest quality is linked to increased signs of aging, a lower life expectancy, pores and skin barrier function.

- **Diet**

Some research shows that eating a diet plan high in glucose and refined carbs can damage the skin over time.

- **Alcoholic beverages and caffeine intake**

Alcohol consumption excessively dehydrates the body. As time passes, this dehydration can cause your skin layer to sag and lose its form.

Caffeine may have an similar impact, although there's conflicting research about if daily espresso consumption causes lines and wrinkles.

- **Environment**

Pigment areas and lines and wrinkles can be triggered or worsened by environmental contaminants.

Since your epidermis makes a direct connection with the environment around you, your skin layer barrier has been put through the toxins and contaminants in your environment.

- **Stress**

A stressful life can result in an inflammatory response within you, as well as harm your sleep practices. Stress hormones and inflammation can age the body faster.

# Chapter 5

## Signs of premature aging

Growing older looks different for everybody, but there are specific signs of aging that are believed "premature" if you see them before you turn 35.

- **Sunspots**

Sunspots, also known as age spots and liver spots, are flat spots on your skin layer caused by many years of sun exposure.

These hyper-pigmented spots may develop on your face, the back of the hands, or your forearms. They have a tendency to appear at or after age 40. People who have fairer pores and skin, like Fitzpatrick type 1 and 2, could see these sun place developments earlier.

- **Gaunt hands**

Over time, the very best layers of your skin layer become thinner and contain fewer structuring proteins, such as collagen, that provide your skin layer its shape.

The hands may begin to appear more veiny, thin, and susceptible to wrinkles because of this. There's no goal metric for when hands begin looking older, but most people have a tendency to notice it throughout their past due to 30s and premature 40s.

- **Inflammation of hyperpigmentation along the chest**

Many people develop patchy discoloration on the chest as they grow older. Much like sunspots, these regions of different pigments can be caused by harm to your cells from direct sun exposure.

This sort of hyperpigmentation isn't always linked to aging. It could be the consequence of eczema or other epidermis conditions that harm the melanin cellular material in your skin layer. There isn't the average age of when this condition of the skin typically appears.

- **Dry or itchy skin**

Dry out or itchy pores and skin (xerosis cutis). That's because lose pores and skin is more vulnerable to dehydration. You might notice your skin layer becoming drier and more susceptible to flaking as you get close to your 40s.

- **Wrinkles or sagging**

As you enter your 30s, your skin layer decreases its creation of collagen, the proteins that give your skin layer its form. Collagen is what helps your skin layer bounce back again and stay plump.

With less collagen in your skin, it's easier for noticeable wrinkles and sagging that occur. You may notice this occurring more in areas around commonly used muscles, like the forehead, or where you're more subjected to the sunlight. The age when people first notice wrinkles vary, with the little standard for when it's "premature." And sometimes aging might not even be responsible. It might simply be dirt or dehydration.

- Hair loss

Hair loss happens as the stem cells that trigger new hair growth in your hair roots die off. Hormonal changes, environmental factors, genetics, as well as your diet all are likely involved in how quickly this happens.

Up to 40 percent of women over age group 70 experience hair loss. Men experience it previously, with 50 percent experiencing hair loss after age group 50.

# What can be done

Once you see the signals of aging, you may take steps to handle the way the body is changing or allow the signs to take its course.

There isn't the right or wrong way to the age, and whatever you decide to pursue with the body is completely your decision.

- **When you have sunspots**

In the event that you notice sunspots, begin by seeing a dermatologist rule out other skin conditions. Knowing for certain what you're working with, think about what lifestyle changes you may make.

Wear sunscreen with at least 30 SPF daily to safeguard yourself from Ultraviolet rays, and reduce immediate exposure to sunlight whenever you can. Covering up when you are outside can assist in preventing further places from appearing.

You may even try treating the sunspots topically to see if indeed they fade. Aloe vera, vitamin C, and products that contain alpha hydroxyl acidity can help treat sunspots.

If those aren't effective, clinical treatment for sunspots includes extreme pulsed light therapy, cryotherapy, and chemical peels.

- **When you have gaunt hands**

If the hands look like gaunt, with translucent, fragile skin and noticeable blood vessels, start moisturizing them regularly. It might be time for you to get one of these new products that cusea hydration directly into your skin. You may even want to use sunscreen with at least 30 SPF to the hands.

If the hands are regularly subjected to chemicals and pollutants through the task that you do or your household chores, it could not be possible to prevent your contact with those ideas completely. Instead, make small changes like putting on gloves when you wash the laundry or weed your garden.

If you're worried about how the hands look, talk with a dermatologist. Clinical treatments for hands include chemical peels, dermal fillers, and laser skin treatment.

- **When you have inflammation or hyperpigmentation**

Whenever you have staining on your upper body, start protecting that part of the body from sunlight whenever possible. Use sunscreen with at least 30 SPF every day, and pay attention to within the parts of your skin layer which have been damaged.

Moisturize the region frequently and look for a lotion with vitamin C or retinoids. You will find products or a doctor can prescribe to take care of hyperpigmentation in your chest area. Mild steroids and bleaching brokers can fade the appearance of hyperpigmentation as time passes.

- **When you have dry or itchy skin**

If your skin layer is flaky, dry, and itchy, you might consult with a dermatologist and eliminate any other health issues. Knowing that dry skin is an indicator of aging rather than an indicator of another thing, start concentrating on lifestyle factors.

Drink more water to keep hydrated during your body as well as your epidermis. Take shorter showers using lukewarm water. See whether the dryness is because of your skin type or if it's actually dehydrated, as the treatments for both differ.

Then find a moisturizer that works for you and use it daily. If turning up your program at home doesn't work, talk with a doctor in regards to a prescription moisturizer that has more powerful elements for protecting your skin layer.

- **When you have lines and wrinkles or sagging skin**

If your skin layer is sagging or you see wrinkles, there are a number of things you are able to do. Begin by protecting your skin layer every day with a sunscreen with at least 30 SPF. Limit your sunlight exposure by putting on hats with a brim and lose clothing that covers your limbs.

If you smoke cigarettes, quitting can assist in preventing further skin damage. Drink water and moisturize your skin each day. Makeup products with green tea extracts, vitamin A, vitamin C, retinoids, and antioxidants may help.

If you'd prefer to go the clinical path, techniques like Botox and dermal fillers can make your skin appear less wrinkled and fuller or lifted.

- **When you have hair loss**

In case your hair is falling out in clumps or growing thinner, consider investing in a shampoo and conditioner product designed to address the problem. Ensure that your diet is filled with nutritious food that nourishes hair. Consider adding a multivitamin or vitamins to help the body make keratin.

Products for hair loss will vary for cisgender women and men. Rogaine (minoxidil) and Propecia (finasteride) are popular over-the-counter treatments.

# Could it be reversed?

You can't stop aging completely and that's a very important thing. Experiences include age, and periodically the skin we have or the body will reflect that. With regards to slowing the indicators you don't like, it's about prevention and providing your cells a lift through products or changes in lifestyle.

In some instances, caring for your skin makes it possible for a healing up process that restores a few of your skin's appearance and restores a little of its structure.

# Preventing further aging

Many factors affect how noticeable your signals of Aging will be. Some you can control, and some you cannot.

- **Use sunscreen**

Putting on sunscreen with at least SPF 30 everyday may be the largest thing you are able to do to prevent signs of premature Aging.

- **Focus on more than simply your face**

Don't limit your moisturizing and skin-protecting routine to just your face. Be sure to use a sunscreen with at least 30 SPF and cream on the other part of the body, too.

Introduce one new product at the same time and give it time for it to work. Some products make significant statements for slowing the symptoms of aging immediately. The simple truth is that any aesthetic product will need some time before you should see noticeable results.

- **Be sure you remove all make-up before bed**

Your face-washing habits can influence just how your skin layer appears. Wash twice each day using tepid to warm water and a mild cleanser. Ensure that your face is free from the basis and other residues prior to going to bed.

- **Adhere to a sleep schedule**

Sleep is vital to all or any organ of the body, iincluding your skin. Following a sleep/rest schedule gives your skin time to renew and renew it daily.

- **Eat a balanced diet**

A balanced diet means that you get every part of the nutrition the body must take in to produce healthy pores and skin cells.

- **Stay hydrated**

Dehydration can make lines and wrinkles arrive faster. Drink 8 glassse of water each day to hydrate the body.

- **Get active**

Daily exercise increases your circulation, which will keep skin healthier. This may help your skin look younger.

- **Stop smoking**

In the event that you stop exposing your skin to the harmful toxins in tobacco smoke, you'll give your skin time to correct. At least one older study from a Trusted Source discovered that participants who stop smoking pointed out that their epidermis looked younger after quitting.

# Chapter 6

## Physical Changes that include Aging

### 1. Heart

The heart pumps all day long and night, whether you are awake or sleeping. It will pump more than 2.5 billion beats throughout your lifetime! As you age, arteries lose their elasticity, fatty debris build-up against artery wall and the cardiovascular must work harder to circulate the blood through the body. These can lead to high blood pressure (hypertension) and atherosclerosis (hardening of the arteries).

Caring for the body with the right type of oil can help you keep the heart healthy and strong. You are able to care for your heart by working out and eating heart-healthy foods.

### 2. Bone fragments, Muscles & Joints

Even as we age, our bone fragments shrink in proportions and density. Some individuals actually become shorter! Others are more susceptible to fractures because of bone reduction. Muscles, tendons, and bones may lose power and flexibility.

Exercise is a superb way to slow or avoid problems with bone fragments, muscles, and joint parts. Maintaining power and flexibility can help keep you strong. Furthermore, a healthy diet plan including calcium can help your bone strong. Make sure to speak to your doctor about what types of exercise and diet are best for you.

**3. Digestive System**

Swallowing and digestive reflexes decelerate as we age. Swallowing could become harder as the oesophagus react less forcefully. The circulation of secretions that help break down food in the belly, liver organ, pancreas, and small intestine can also be reduced. The reduced movement may lead to digestive conditions that weren't present when you were more youthful.

**4. Kidneys and Urinary System**

Kidneys could become less efficient in removing waste materials from the blood because your kidneys get smaller as they lose cellular material as you age. Chronic diseases such as diabetes or high blood pressure can cause even more harm to kidneys.

Urinary incontinence might occur credited to a number of health issues. Changes in hormone quantity in women and having an enlarged prostate in men are adding factors that lead to bladder control problems.

## 5. Brain and Nervous System

Once we age, we naturally lose cellular material. That is even true in the mind. Memory reduction occurs because the number of brain cellular material decreases. The heart can compensate because of this reduction by increasing the number of connections between cellular materials to protect brain function. Reflexes may decelerate, distraction is much more likely and coordination is affected.

## 6. Eyes

There are several vision changes that occur even as we age. We might need help viewing items that are nearer as our zoom lens stiffens. We might have a far more difficult time viewing in low-light conditions, and colors may be recognized differently. Our eye may be less with the capacity of producing tears and our lens could become cloudier.

Common eye problems associated with age include cataracts, glaucoma, and macular degeneration.

## 7. Ears

Excessive noise during your lifetime can cause hearing loss as you age. Many old adults have a problem hearing higher-pitched voices and noises, trouble hearing in occupied places and more often accumulating earwax.

## 8. Hair, Pores and skin, and Nails

As you age, your skin layer becomes drier and brittle, which can result in more lines and wrinkles. The fat coating under your skin thins, which leads to less sweating. This might seem just like a positive thing, but it certainly makes you more vulnerable to temperature stroke and high temperature exhaustion in the summertime. Hair and fingernails grow slower and are brittle. The hair will slim and turn grey.

## 9. Weight

Decreasing degrees of exercise and a slowing metabolism may donate to weight gain. The body might not have the ability to burn as much calorie consumption as it once could, and the ones extra calorie consumption will finish up being stockpiled as fat.

When you can't prevent aging, you can get ready for the many effects of aging, both inside and outside the body.

# Anti-Aging Foods to support Your 40s and Beyond Body

Whenever we pack our diet with vibrant foods packed with antioxidants, healthy fats, drinking water, and essential nutrients, the body will show its appreciation through its largest organ: the skin we have. In the end, your skin is usually the first part of the body to show inner trouble, and there's only a lot that lotions, lotions, masks, and serums can do before we have to take a nearer look at what's fuelling us.

Experts have even concluded that eating fruits and vegetables is the safest and healthiest way to fight dull complexions and fine lines. Prepared to shine? Listed below are 10 of the greatest anti-aging foods to nourish the body for a shine that originates from within.

## 1. Watercress

The health advantages of watercress don't disappoint! This nutrient-dense hydrating leafy green is a superb way to obtain:

- Calcium.

- Potassium.

- Manganese.

- Phosphorus.

- nutritional vitamins A, C, K, B-1, and B-2

Watercress functions as an interior pore and skin antiseptic and escalates the blood circulation and delivery of minerals Trusted Source to all or any cells of your body, resulting in improved oxygenation of your skin. Packed with nutritional vitamins A and C, the antioxidants in watercress Trusted Source may neutralize dangerous free radicals, assisting to keep fine lines and lines and wrinkles away.

**To try**: Put in a couple of this flavourful green to your salad today for glowing epidermis and overall improved health!

OTHER YOUTHFUL BENEFITS

This delicious green could also boost immunity Trusted Source (as observed in trouts), aid digestion (in a single cell study), and offer thyroid support because of its iodine content.

## 2. Red bell pepper

Red bell peppers contain antioxidants Trusted Source which reign supreme as it pertains to anti-aging. Furthermore, with their high content of vitamin C which is wonderful for collagen creation, red bell peppers contain powerful antioxidants called carotenoids.

Carotenoids are herb pigments accountable for the scarlet, yellow, and orange colors you observe in many fruits & vegetables. They have a number of anti-inflammatory properties Trusted Source and could help protect pores and skin from sunlight damage Trusted Source, air pollution, and environmental harmful toxins.

**To try:** Cut bell peppers and dip them in hummus as a treat, add them into a raw salad, or cook them up in a stir-fry.

## 3. Papaya

This delicious superfood is abundant with a number of

antioxidants, vitamins, and minerals that might help to improve Trusted Source skin elasticity and minimize the looks of fine lines and wrinkles. Included in these are:

- nutritional vitamins A, C, K, and E

- calcium

- potassium

- magnesium

- phosphorus

- B vitamins

The wide selection of antioxidants in papaya really helps to fight free radical harm and may hold off signs of aging Trusted Source. Papaya also includes an enzyme called papain, which gives additional anti-aging benefits by working as nature's best anti-inflammatory brokers. It's also within many exfoliating products.

So yes, eating papaya (or using products containing papain) can help the body shed dead epidermis cellular material, leaving you with glowing, vibrant pores and skin!

**To try:** Drizzle fresh lime juice over a large bowl of papaya in your breakfast or make a papaya mask at home for the next night in!

## 4. Blueberries

Blueberries are abundant with nutritional vitamins A and C, as well as an age-defying antioxidant called anthocyanin. This is exactly what provides blueberries their deep, beautiful blue color.

These powerful antioxidants Trusted Source can help protect skin from harm because of the sun, stress, and pollution by moderating the inflammatory response and avoiding collagen loss Trusted Source.

**To try:** Toss this great-tasting, low-sugar fruit into an early morning smoothie or fruit dish, and allow it to give a beautifying punch!

## 5. Broccoli

Broccoli can be an anti-inflammatory, anti-aging powerhouse filled with:

- nutritional vitamins C and K

- a number of antioxidants

- fiber

- folate

- lutein

- calcium

The body needs vitamin C for the creation of collagen, the primary protein in the epidermis that provides its strength and elasticity.

- To try: You are able to eat broccoli raw for an instant treat, but if you have enough time, softly steam before eating. From charred bites to pesto sauces, cooking food broccoli actually helps release more health advantages for the body.

### *Other Youthful Benefits*

The nutrient lutein has been linked Trusted Source to the preservation of the brain's memory function, as well as vitamin K and calcium (which are crucial for bone health insurance and preventing osteoporosis). Will there be anything this anti-aging cruciferous veggie can't do?

## 6. Spinach

Spinach is super hydrating and filled with antioxidants that help oxygenate and replenish the whole body. It's also abundant with:

- nutritional vitamins A, C, Electronic, and K

- magnesium

- plant-based heme iron

- lutein

This versatile leafy green's high vitamin C content enhances collagen production to keep skin firm and smooth. But that's not absolutely all. Vitamin A it offers may promote strong, gleaming hair, while vitamin K has been shown Trusted Source in reducing inflammation in cellular material.

- To try: Add handfuls of spinach to a smoothie, salad, or sautéé. More ideas? Have a look at well-known spinach quality recipes, including spinach potato chips and cheesy burgers.

## 7. Nuts

Many nuts (especially almonds) are a great way to obtain vitamin E, which might help repair skin tissue, retain skin moisture, and protect skin from harmful Ultraviolet rays. Walnuts even contain Trusted Source anti-inflammatory omega-3 essential fatty acids that might help:

- strengthen skin cell membranes

- protect against sunlight damage

- give skin a lovely shine by preserving its natural oil barrier

**To try**: Sprinkle a variety of nuts together with your salads, or eat a few as a treat. Don't take away the pores and skin, either, as studies also show that 50 percent or more Trusted Way to obtain the antioxidants are lost without your skin.

EATING Nut products

• reduced risk for cardiovascular disease (walnuts) and

type 2 diabetes (pistachios)

•potential prevention of cognitive decrease in old adults (almonds)

## 8. Avocado

Avocados are saturated in inflammation-fighting essential fatty acids that promote clean, supple skin. In addition, they include a variety of essential nutrition that may avoid the unwanted effects of aging Trusted Source, including:

- nutritional vitamins K, C, Electronic, and A

- B vitamins

- potassium

The high content of vitamin A in avocados can help us shed deceased skin cells, departing us with gorgeous, glowing skin. Their carotenoid content could also assist in obstructing toxins and harm from the sun's rays and also help protect against epidermis cancers.

To try: Toss some avocado into a salad, smoothie, or

simply eat it with a spoon. Just when you thought you've attempted all the ways to consume an avocado, we've got 23 more. You can even check it out topically as an unbelievable moisturizing face mask to fight to swell, reduce inflammation, and assist in preventing wrinkles!

## 9. Sweet potatoes

The orange color of the  potato originates from an antioxidant called beta-carotene which is changed into vitamin A. Vitamin A Trusted Source can help restore pores and skin elasticity, promote epidermis cellular turnover and eventually contribute to smooth, youthful-looking pores and skin.

This delicious root vegetable is also a great way to obtain vitamins C and E both which may protect the skin we have from harmful free radicals and keep our complexion radiant.

**To try:** Make one of the sweet potato toast recipes that will up your breakfast or treat the game like no other. Thanksgiving isn't the only time to include this veggie to your daily diet!

## 10. Pomegranate seeds

Pomegranates have been used for years and years as a recovery medicinal fruit. Saturated in vitamin C and a number of powerful antioxidants Trusted Source, pomegranates may protect the body from free radical harm and reduce degrees of inflammation inside our system.

These healthy fruits also include a compound called punicalagin, which might help preserve collagen in your skin, slowing signs of aging.

**To try:** Sprinkle these sweet little jewels onto an infant spinach walnut salad for an anti-aging treat!

OTHER YOUTHFUL BENEFITS

Research, in addition, has shown a substance called urolithin A Trusted Source, which is produced when pomegranates connect to gut bacteria, may rejuvenate mitochondria. It had been even seen to invert muscle aging Trusted Source in rat studies.

Flood the body with powerful nutrients

By nourishing ourselves with these anti-aging foods, we can gain gas to appear and feel our best. If you're looking to get more mouth-watering vegetation to try, choose vegetables & fruits deep in color. The wealthy shades generally are a signal of more powerful radical fighting capabilities to keep your skin layer healthy and lively. The greater colors you can fit on your dish, the better.

# Chapter 7

## Anti-Aging Natural herbs: 8 Ayurveda Herbal products To Decelerate Aging

Aging can be inevitable; it entails the changes in a person with physical, mental, mental and public change. Wrinkled pores and skin, greying hair and macular degeneration are a few symptoms of Aging. While one cannot avoid these charges, but will surely hold them off through medications, natural kitchen substances or Ayurvedic natural herbs. Ayurveda may be the artwork of daily residing in tranquility and laws and regulations of nature. It really is a historical natural knowledge of health insurance and recovery. Ayurvedic treatment for a disease is targeted on three doshas of the person - Vata dosha, Kapha dosha, and pitta dosha. It feels in keeping a perfect balance among these three aspects, which is the trick to staying younger and healthy. The procedure of degenerating cells as you get old is recognized as Aging. Ayurveda suggests herbal products that will help decrease the symptoms of Aging by regenerating cells. A lot of the herbal remedies have various antioxidants that inhibit the development of cells harming free radicals in the torso. Relating to Ayurveda expert from Nirog Street, Ram memory N Kumar, "Rasayana (rejuvenation) branch of Ayurveda specifically handles Aging and its own results. Aging is a degenerative and palliative stage and process, Rasayana inspections speed and impact considerably, resulting in deceleration. Rasayana treatment is preferred to folks who are 35 years of age and more."

**Suggested Herbs that can be eaten to delay Aging**
**Guduchi**

Guduchi, or Giloy, may revive the skin we have tissues and handle inflamed epidermis conditions by its anti-inflammatory properties. Guduchi is accountable for promoting mental clearness and enhance our disease fighting capability.

**2. Guggulu**

Guggulu is a robust and potent herb that comes from the flowering tree Mukul Myrrh. Its anti-inflammatory properties assist in combating various diseases and inhibit the development of free radicals in the torso.

## 3. Brahmi

Brahmi, or Bacopa, is a memory enhancer, especially useful for individuals who may be experiencing age-related memory reduction. It is thought to have refreshing results on the human brain.

## 4. Amalaki

Amalaki, or Amla, is a great way to obtain Vitamin-C and antioxidants that help the body battle various diseases. Also, it can help you remain safe from age-related macular degeneration and Cataract.

## 5. Turmeric

The compound curcumin in Turmeric possesses a robust anti-Aging effect. They have anti-inflammatory properties and antioxidants that help to keep diseases away.

## 6. Ginseng

Ginseng contains a lot of phytochemicals that help stimulate and activate the skin's metabolism. These phytochemicals also help you to get gone free radicals that get gathered when your epidermis is subjected to pollution and sunshine.

**7. Gotu-kola**

Gotu kola is abundant with flavonoids with antioxidant activity that helps protect your skin and body which makes it an exceptionally essential anti-Aging herb.

**8. Ashwagandha**

Ashwagandha assists with rapid cellular regeneration and rejuvenation that subsequently assists with delaying signals of Aging, especially regarding the skin.

Be sure you use these herbs under the supervision of the Ayurvedic expert. Get older, don't age!

# Best Anti-Aging Herbs for Youthful Skin

### 1. Basil

Holy basil or tulsi assists with preventing the signals of aging. Extreme UV exposure on the skin layer causes collagen depletion. Collagen is the substance that maintains the elasticity of your skin layer. In a report, researchers discovered that topical software of basil helped in keeping skin dampness quantity, reduced pores and skin roughness and scales, avoided lines and wrinkles, and made your skin smooth.

**How to Use Basil For Anti-Aging Benefits**

**YOU'LL NEED**

- 1 cup holy basil leaves

- 1 tablespoon gram flour

- 1 teaspoon honey

**Method**

- Soak the basil leaves in hot water to soften them and make a paste.

- Blend it with gram flour and honey.

- Use it to that person and allow it dry.

- Clean with lukewarm drinking water.

**2. Cinnamon**

Cinnamon is trusted in Ayurvedic medication for its recovery properties. Additionally, it is thought to have anti-aging benefits as it prevents collagen breaks down and prevents a lack of epidermis elasticity. A report says it also increases collagen synthesis and prevents indicators of Aging.

## How to Use Cinnamon For Anti-Aging Benefits

### YOU'LL NEED

- 1 teaspoon cinnamon powder

- 1 tablespoon natural honey

### Method

- Mix both ingredients.

- Apply the facial skin mask.

- Leave it on for 10-15 minutes.

- Clean with lukewarm drinking water.

## 3. Clove

Clove has immense health advantages. Clove essential oil

is trusted in Ayurveda for dealing with many ailments. A report has also discovered that clove has free radical scavenging properties that possess antioxidants that decelerate signs of Aging.

**How to Use Clove For Anti-Aging Benefits**

**YOU'LL NEED**

- 1 tablespoon coconut oil

- 3-4 drops clove oil

**Method**

- Wash that person with tepid to warm water (you can also steam it a little).

- Combine the coconut and clove natural oils.

- Massage on that person and allow it to stay for around 30 minutes.

- Wash that person with cool water.

**4. Ginger**

This herb has been found in Ayurvedic and Chinese

medicine for over a large number of years for treating multiple ailments. Ginger has high degrees of antioxidants and anti-inflammatory properties that assist in preventing the signs of aging. A report discovered that ginger could control the creation of dangerous free radicals that have an effect on your metabolism and increase oxidative stress, which is bad for your skin layer.

**How to Use Ginger For Anti-Aging Benefits**

**YOU'LL NEED**

- 2 tablespoons essential olive oil

- 4 tablespoons brown sugar

- 1 tablespoon grated ginger

**Method**

- Clean your skin layer with a moderate cleanser.

- Blend all the elements.

- Scrub that person with the mixture for ten minutes.

- Leave it on for another 5-10 minutes.

- Clean it off with lukewarm drinking water.

## 5. Guggulu

Guggulu is an extremely powerful plant that is extracted from the Mukul Myrrh tree. A report discovered that Guggula could prevent lines and wrinkles. Additionally, it is used because of its anti-inflammatory properties that inhibit the result of the dangerous free radicals.

**How to Use Guggula For Anti-Aging Benefits**

**YOU'LL NEED**

- 1 teaspoon Guggula powder

- 1 tablespoon coconut essential oil (or shea butter)

**Method**

- Mix the natural powder with essential oil or butter.

- Massage the combination on that person (use it as a night time cream).

- Let it stick to overnight.

- Clean it off the very next day.

# 6. Gingko

It is one herb that is widely studied because of its immense health advantages. Gingko Biloba is revered because of its memory space improving properties, but additionally, it is known because of its anti-aging benefits. A medical study discovered that Gingko components, when applied on pores and skin, could prevent lines and wrinkles and enhance skin consistency by increasing hydration and epidermis smoothness and reducing roughness.

## How to Use Gingko For Anti-Aging Benefits

## YOU'LL NEED

- 1 teaspoon Gingko extract

- 1 tablespoon bentonite clay

- 1 tablespoon honey

## Method

- Mix the clay-based and honey and make a paste.

- If the regularity is too thick, use distilled drinking

water.

- Combine the Gingko extracts with the pack.

- Use it to that person. Let it dried out.

- Clean with lukewarm drinking water.

## 7. Ashwagandha

Ashwagandha or Indian ginseng or winter cherry can be an extremely popular natural herb used because of its medicinal properties. They have antibacterial, antifungal, and cognitive enhancing properties and it is packed with alkaloids that protect the cellular material (including skin cellular material) from oxidative stress and harm. This keeps your skin layer healthy and the symptoms of aging away.

**How to Use Ashwagandha For Anti-Aging Benefits**

**YOU'LL NEED**

- ½ teaspoon ashwagandha powder

- ½ teaspoon dried out ginger powder

- ½ teaspoon lemon juice (diluted)

**Method**

- Blend all the substances and make a paste.

- Add a little water if it's too thick.

- Apply everything over that person and allow it dry.

- Clean it off with drinking water.

## 8. Ginseng

This Chinese medicinal herb is popular worldwide because of its anti-aging benefits. A report found that an assortment of ginseng and Chinese language hawthorn protected your skin from the consequences of Aging. It boosts procollagen synthesis and wetness quantity of your skin and prevents wrinkle development.

**How to Use Ginseng For Anti-Aging Benefits**

**YOU'LL NEED**

- 1 teaspoon ginseng powder

- 1 cup hot water

- Cotton balls

**Method**

- Combine the ginseng natural powder in water.

- Allow it cool.

- Soak the natural cotton ball in the toner and apply everything over that person and neck.

- Leave it on overnight.

- Wash off the very next day with tepid to warm water.

## 9. Horlistail

Also known as shave grass or mare's tail, this perennial herb contains natural silicon that can provide you youthful and glowing pore and skin. Horlistail includes flavonoids, vitamins Electronic and C, carotenoids, and coenzyme Q10 that enhance the collagen quantity in your skin layer, neutralize the dangerous free radicals, and improve the epidermis firmness.

# How to Use Horlistail for Anti-Aging Benefits

**YOU'LL NEED**

- 1 tablespoon chopped horsetail shoot

- 3 tablespoons uncooked honey

**Method**

- Warm the honey and blend the horsetail take in it.

- Store it for 2-3 times and then stress the honey.

- Consume a tablespoon of any risk of strain twice per day.

## 10. Oregano

This herb not only makes your meal taste good, but it additionally helps in slowing the aging of your skin layer. Oregano is a storehouse of antioxidants and flavonoids that prevent free radical harm and hold off the signals of Aging.

**How to Use Oregano for Anti-Aging Benefits**

**YOU'LL NEED**

- 10-15 drops oregano gas

- 2 tablespoons olive, coconut, or jojoba oil

**Method**

- Mix the fundamental oil with the carrier oil.

- Use the blend for massaging that person and neck.

- Apply before bedtime and keep it on immediately.

- Wash off the very next day.

## 11. Rosemary

This herb protects your skin layer from photodamage. Extreme exposure to Ultraviolet rays causes fine lines, lines and wrinkles, and other indicators of UV-induced Aging. Rosemary prevents photodamage while enhancing your skin's elasticity and stopping lines and wrinkles.

**How to Use Rosemary for Anti-Aging Benefits**

**YOU'LL NEED**

- 2 cups of water

- 2 fresh sprigs of rosemary

- 3 tablespoons apple cider vinegar

**Method**

- Combine all the elements in a container and boil it on medium warmth.

- Simmer for some time (before the number is reduced to fifty percent) and allow it cool.

- Strain the water and store it in an aerosol bottle.

- Use it as a toner for your skin layer.

## 12. Sage

Sage is abundant with antioxidants that assist in reversing the signs of Aging, such as age spots, lines and wrinkles, and fine lines. Sage consists of flavonoids, phenolic carboxylic acids, phenolic diterpenes, and other antioxidants that protect your skin layer from Aging.

**How to Use Sage for Anti-Aging Benefits**

**YOU'LL NEED**

- 1 ½ teaspoons sage leaves

- 1 cup of water

**Method**

- Boil sage leaves in a skillet filled with drinking water and steep it for 20-30 minutes.

- Strain the water and allow it to cool down.

- Transfer it to a cup bottle and use it as a toner.

### 13. Thyme

That is another herb with multiple benefits. It not only makes your meal flavorful but also prevents skin surface damage and symptoms of Aging. Thyme is free of charge radical scavenger and has antioxidant and anti-inflammatory properties that protect your skin layer from the signals of Aging.

**How to Use Thyme for Anti-Aging Benefits**

**YOU'LL NEED**

- 1 tablespoon dried thyme

- ½ cup alcohol-free witch hazel

**Method**

- Take a cup jar and add the substances to it.

- Allow thyme soak in the witch hazel for weekly.

- Stress it and then use it as a toner.

## 14. Gotu Kola

In Ayurveda, Gotukola is known as a magic treatment because of its Vayasthapana (meaning age-defying properties). The Ayurvedic text messages say that it keeps a balance between all the doshas within you and promotes collagen synthesis.

# How to Use Gotukola for Anti-Aging Benefits

## *You'll Need*

- A small number of dried Gotu kola

- A small number of calendula plants (optionally available)

- Sesame oil (you may use coconut, olive, jojoba, or almond oil)

- A glass jar

## Method

- Place the herbs into the cup jar and put oil involved with it.

- Ensure that the oil addresses the herbs completely.

- Fasten the lid and tremble the jar a little.

- Allow it infuse for 2-3 several weeks.

- Leave the bottle under sunlight for the duration.

Use it as therapeutic massage oil around the body and face.

CPSIA information can be obtained
at www.ICGtesting.com
Printed in the USA
BVHW041404281220
596561BV00009BA/1662

9 781637 500453